GASTROPARESIS SMOOTHIES COOKBOOK FOR BEGINNER

100 Fruit Blends Recipes for Gastric and Relieving Abdominal Pain.

Michael Samuel

All rights reserved. No part of this work may be reproduced, distributed, or transmitted in any form or by any means, including photocopying, recording, or other electronic or mechanical methods, without the prior written permission of the copyright owner.

TABLE OF CONTENTS

1. INTRODUCTION

Understanding Gastroparesis

Gastroparesis is a condition that affects the stomach muscles and prevents proper stomach emptying. This can lead to symptoms such as nausea, vomiting, bloating, and abdominal pain. Causes of gastroparesis can include diabetes, certain medications, and surgeries that affect the stomach. It is crucial to manage this condition through dietary adjustments and medical treatment to improve quality of life.

Benefits of Smoothies for Gastroparesis

Smoothies can be an excellent dietary option for those with gastroparesis due to their smooth texture and easy digestibility. The key benefits of smoothies include:

- - Easy Digestion: Blended fruits and vegetables are easier on the stomach and can help alleviate symptoms.

- - Nutrient-Rich: Smoothies can be packed with essential vitamins, minerals, and antioxidants.
- - Hydration: They provide fluids that are crucial for maintaining hydration, especially if solid food intake is limited.
- - Customization: Ingredients can be tailored to meet individual nutritional needs and preferences.

Essential Ingredients and Their Benefits

Choosing the right ingredients is vital for making gastroparesis-friendly smoothies. Here are some beneficial ingredients:

- - Fruits: Bananas, berries, apples, and pears provide essential nutrients and are generally easy to digest.
- - Vegetables: Spinach, kale, and cucumber add fiber and vitamins without adding heaviness.
- - Liquids: Water, coconut water, and almond milk keep smoothies light and hydrating.

- - Additives: Ginger aids digestion, aloe vera soothes the digestive tract, and turmeric has anti-inflammatory properties.

Tips for Making Smoothies Easier to Digest

To maximize the benefits of smoothies and ensure they are gentle on the stomach, consider the following tips:

- - Blending Techniques: Blend ingredients thoroughly to achieve a smooth, lump-free consistency.
- - Portion Sizes: Keep portions small to prevent overwhelming the stomach.
- - Digestive Aids: Incorporate ingredients like ginger and peppermint to aid digestion.
- - Timing and Frequency: Consume smaller, more frequent servings rather than large amounts at once to avoid discomfort.

2. GETTING STARTED

Tools and Equipment

To create delicious and nutritious smoothies, you'll need the right tools and equipment:

- - Blender: A high-quality blender is essential for achieving a smooth consistency. Consider a powerful blender if you plan to blend tougher ingredients like kale or frozen fruit.
- - Measuring Cups and Spoons: Accurate measurements help maintain consistency in flavor and texture.
- - Cutting Board and Knife: For preparing fruits and vegetables before blending.
- - Spatula: Useful for scraping down the sides of the blender to ensure all ingredients are well mixed.
- - Storage Containers: Glass jars or BPA-free plastic containers for storing leftover smoothies.

Basic Techniques for Smoothie Preparation

Creating the perfect smoothie involves a few basic techniques:

- - Layering Ingredients: Add liquids first, followed by soft ingredients like yogurt or bananas, then greens, and finally frozen items. This layering helps the blender work efficiently.
- - Blending in Stages: Start on a low speed to chop up the ingredients, then gradually increase to a higher speed for a smooth finish.
- - Adjusting Consistency: If the smoothie is too thick, add more liquid. If it's too thin, add more fruit or yogurt.
- - Balancing Flavors: Experiment with different combinations to find a balance between sweet, tart, and creamy elements.

Storing and Serving Smoothies

Proper storage and serving practices can enhance the smoothie experience:

- - Immediate Consumption: For the best texture and nutritional value, consume smoothies immediately after preparation.
- - Refrigeration: If you need to store a smoothie, keep it in an airtight container in the refrigerator for up to 24 hours. Shake well before drinking.
- - Freezing: Smoothies can be frozen in individual portions. Thaw in the refrigerator overnight or blend briefly to restore the texture.
- - Serving Ideas: Serve smoothies in a chilled glass or bowl. Garnish with fresh fruit, nuts, or seeds for added texture and nutrition.

Safety and Hygiene

Maintaining safety and hygiene is crucial when preparing smoothies:

- - Washing Produce: Always wash fruits and vegetables thoroughly to remove dirt and pesticides.

- - Handling Equipment: Clean blenders and utensils immediately after use to prevent bacterial growth.
- - Food Safety: Use fresh ingredients and check expiration dates on packaged items. Discard any ingredients that show signs of spoilage.
- - Allergy Awareness: Be mindful of potential allergens in ingredients, especially if serving others. Clearly label any smoothies that contain common allergens like nuts or dairy.

3. FOUNDATION RECIPES

Basic Smoothie Bases

Creating a versatile smoothie base is essential for building various recipes. Here are a few foundational smoothie bases to get you started:

1. Banana Base
- 1 ripe banana
- 1 cup of almond milk (or any preferred milk)
- ½ cup of plain yogurt

2. Berry Base
- 1 cup of mixed berries (fresh or frozen)
- 1 cup of coconut water
- ½ cup of Greek yogurt

3. Green Base
- 1 cup of spinach or kale
- 1 apple, cored and sliced
- 1 cup of water or green tea

4. Tropical Base
- 1 cup of pineapple chunks
- ½ mango, peeled and diced
- 1 cup of coconut milk

Choosing the Right Liquids

The choice of liquid can significantly affect the taste and texture of your smoothie. Here are some options and their benefits:

1. Water
- Neutral flavor
- Keeps the smoothie light and hydrating

2. Coconut Water
- Naturally sweet
- Rich in electrolytes, great for hydration

3. Almond Milk
- Mild, nutty flavor
- Low in calories and dairy-free

4. Coconut Milk

- Creamy texture
- Adds a tropical flavor and is dairy-free

5. Greek Yogurt
- Thick and creamy
- High in protein and probiotics

6. Fruit Juice
- Adds sweetness and flavor
- Use in moderation due to high sugar content

7. Green Tea
- Light, earthy flavor
- Contains antioxidants and a mild caffeine boost

Sweeteners and Flavor Enhancers

Enhancing the flavor of your smoothies can make them more enjoyable and nutritious. Here are some sweeteners and flavor enhancers to consider:

1. Honey

- Natural sweetener with antibacterial properties
- Use sparingly to avoid excess sugar

2. Maple Syrup
- Adds a rich, earthy sweetness
- Great for adding depth of flavor

3. Stevia
- Calorie-free natural sweetener
- Ideal for those managing sugar intake

4. Vanilla Extract
- Adds a warm, sweet aroma and flavor
- Enhances the taste without adding sugar

5. Cinnamon
- Adds warmth and a slight sweetness
- Can help regulate blood sugar levels

6. Ginger
- Adds a spicy kick and aids digestion
- Use fresh or powdered ginger

7. Mint

- Fresh, cooling flavor
- Pairs well with fruits like watermelon and berries

8. Lemon or Lime Juice

- Adds a zesty, refreshing tang
- Balances sweetness and adds brightness to flavors

Experiment with these bases, liquids, and enhancers to create your unique smoothie recipes that cater to your taste preferences and nutritional needs.

4. FRUIT SMOOTHIES

Banana and Berry Bliss

Ingredients:
- 1 ripe banana
- 1 cup mixed berries (strawberries, blueberries, raspberries)
- 1 cup almond milk
- ½ cup Greek yogurt
- 1 tablespoon honey (optional)

Instructions:
1. Place the banana, mixed berries, almond milk, and Greek yogurt in a blender.
2. Blend until smooth.
3. Taste and add honey if additional sweetness is desired.
4. Pour into a glass and enjoy immediately.

Tropical Mango Medley

Ingredients:

- 1 cup mango chunks (fresh or frozen)
- ½ cup pineapple chunks
- 1 cup coconut milk
- ½ banana
- 1 tablespoon chia seeds (optional)

Instructions:
1. Add the mango, pineapple, coconut milk, and banana to the blender.
2. Blend until creamy and smooth.
3. If using, add chia seeds and blend briefly to mix.
4. Serve in a chilled glass.

Apple and Pear Fusion

Ingredients:
- 1 apple, cored and chopped
- 1 pear, cored and chopped
- 1 cup spinach (optional for added nutrients)
- 1 cup water or apple juice
- 1 tablespoon lemon juice

Instructions:

1. Place the apple, pear, spinach (if using), water or apple juice, and lemon juice in the blender.
2. Blend until smooth and well combined.
3. Pour into a glass and enjoy the refreshing fusion of flavors.

Melon Melody

Ingredients:
- 1 cup watermelon chunks
- 1 cup cantaloupe chunks
- 1 cup honeydew melon chunks
- ½ cup coconut water
- 1 tablespoon fresh mint leaves

Instructions:
1. Combine the watermelon, cantaloupe, honeydew melon, and coconut water in a blender.
2. Blend until smooth and well mixed.
3. Add the fresh mint leaves and blend briefly to incorporate.
4. Serve immediately in a chilled glass for a cool and refreshing treat.

5. GREEN SMOOTHIES

Spinach and Pineapple Delight

Ingredients:
- 1 cup fresh spinach
- 1 cup pineapple chunks (fresh or frozen)
- 1 banana
- 1 cup coconut water
- 1 tablespoon chia seeds (optional)

Instructions:
1. Add the spinach, pineapple chunks, banana, and coconut water to the blender.
2. Blend until smooth and creamy.
3. If using, add chia seeds and blend briefly to mix.
4. Pour into a glass and enjoy the vibrant green delight.

Kale and Kiwi Combo

Ingredients:

- 1 cup fresh kale leaves, stems removed
- 2 kiwis, peeled and sliced
- 1 banana
- 1 cup orange juice
- 1 tablespoon flaxseeds (optional)

Instructions:

1. Place the kale, kiwis, banana, and orange juice in the blender.
2. Blend until well combined and smooth.
3. If using, add flaxseeds and blend briefly to mix.
4. Serve in a glass and enjoy the nutrient-packed combo.

Cucumber and Melon Cooler

Ingredients:
- 1 cucumber, peeled and chopped
- 1 cup honeydew melon chunks
- 1 cup green grapes
- 1 cup water
- 1 tablespoon fresh mint leaves

Instructions:
1. Combine the cucumber, honeydew melon, green grapes, and water in the blender.
2. Blend until smooth and refreshing.
3. Add the fresh mint leaves and blend briefly to incorporate.
4. Pour into a glass and enjoy the cool, hydrating smoothie.

Avocado and Green Apple Smoothie

Ingredients:
- ½ avocado, peeled and pitted
- 1 green apple, cored and chopped
- 1 cup spinach
- 1 cup almond milk
- 1 tablespoon lemon juice

Instructions:
1. Add the avocado, green apple, spinach, almond milk, and lemon juice to the blender.
2. Blend until creamy and well combined.
3. Serve immediately in a glass and savor the creamy, nutrient-rich smoothie.

6. BERRY SMOOTHIES

Blueberry Banana Blend

Ingredients:
- 1 cup blueberries (fresh or frozen)
- 1 banana
- 1 cup almond milk
- ½ cup Greek yogurt
- 1 tablespoon honey (optional)

Instructions:
1. Place the blueberries, banana, almond milk, and Greek yogurt in a blender.
2. Blend until smooth and creamy.
3. Taste and add honey if additional sweetness is desired.
4. Pour into a glass and enjoy the delicious blend.

Raspberry Peach Smoothie

Ingredients:

- 1 cup raspberries (fresh or frozen)
- 1 peach, pitted and sliced
- 1 cup coconut water
- ½ cup plain yogurt
- 1 teaspoon vanilla extract

Instructions:
1. Add the raspberries, peach, coconut water, plain yogurt, and vanilla extract to the blender.
2. Blend until well combined and smooth.
3. Serve immediately in a chilled glass.

Strawberry Lemonade Smoothie

Ingredients:
- 1 cup strawberries (fresh or frozen)
- 1 banana
- 1 cup lemon juice
- 1 cup water
- 1 tablespoon honey (optional)

Instructions:
1. Combine the strawberries, banana, lemon juice, and water in a blender.

2. Blend until smooth and refreshing.
3. Taste and add honey if additional sweetness is needed.
4. Pour into a glass and enjoy the tangy, sweet smoothie.

Mixed Berry Boost

Ingredients:
- 1 cup mixed berries (strawberries, blueberries, raspberries, blackberries)
- 1 banana
- 1 cup orange juice
- ½ cup Greek yogurt
- 1 tablespoon chia seeds (optional)

Instructions:
1. Place the mixed berries, banana, orange juice, and Greek yogurt in the blender.
2. Blend until smooth and well combined.
3. If using, add chia seeds and blend briefly to mix.
4. Serve immediately in a glass and enjoy the berry-licious boost.

7. CITRUS SMOOTHIES

Orange Creamsicle Smoothie

Ingredients:
- 1 orange, peeled and segmented
- 1 banana
- 1 cup vanilla almond milk (or any preferred milk)
- ½ cup Greek yogurt
- 1 teaspoon vanilla extract
- 1 tablespoon honey (optional)

Instructions:
1. Place the orange, banana, vanilla almond milk, Greek yogurt, and vanilla extract in a blender.
2. Blend until smooth and creamy.
3. Taste and add honey if additional sweetness is desired.
4. Pour into a glass and enjoy the creamy, citrus delight.

Grapefruit and Strawberry Twist

Ingredients:
- 1 grapefruit, peeled and segmented
- 1 cup strawberries (fresh or frozen)
- 1 banana
- 1 cup water
- 1 tablespoon honey (optional)

Instructions:
1. Add the grapefruit, strawberries, banana, and water to the blender.
2. Blend until smooth and well combined.
3. Taste and add honey if additional sweetness is needed.
4. Serve immediately in a glass and enjoy the refreshing twist.

Lemon and Lime Refresher

Ingredients:
- 1 lemon, peeled and seeded
- 1 lime, peeled and seeded
- 1 banana

- 1 cup coconut water
- 1 tablespoon honey (optional)

Instructions:
1. Combine the lemon, lime, banana, and coconut water in a blender.
2. Blend until smooth and refreshing.
3. Taste and add honey if additional sweetness is desired.
4. Pour into a glass and enjoy the zesty, refreshing smoothie.

Tangerine and Mango Tango

Ingredients:
- 2 tangerines, peeled and segmented
- 1 cup mango chunks (fresh or frozen)
- 1 banana
- 1 cup water
- 1 tablespoon chia seeds (optional)

Instructions:
1. Place the tangerines, mango chunks, banana, and water in the blender.

2. Blend until smooth and well combined.
3. If using, add chia seeds and blend briefly to mix.
4. Serve immediately in a glass and enjoy the tropical tango.

8. TROPICAL SMOOTHIES

Pineapple Coconut Dream

Ingredients:
- 1 cup pineapple chunks (fresh or frozen)
- 1 cup coconut milk
- 1 banana
- 1 tablespoon shredded coconut
- 1 teaspoon honey (optional)

Instructions:
1. Add the pineapple chunks, coconut milk, banana, and shredded coconut to the blender.
2. Blend until smooth and creamy.
3. Taste and add honey if additional sweetness is desired.
4. Pour into a glass and enjoy the tropical dream.

Papaya Passion Smoothie

Ingredients:
- 1 cup papaya chunks (fresh or frozen)

- 1 banana
- 1 cup orange juice
- ½ cup Greek yogurt
- 1 tablespoon chia seeds (optional)

Instructions:
1. Combine the papaya chunks, banana, orange juice, and Greek yogurt in the blender.
2. Blend until smooth and well combined.
3. If using, add chia seeds and blend briefly to mix.
4. Serve immediately in a glass and enjoy the passion-filled smoothie.

Coconut Banana Bliss

Ingredients:
- 1 banana
- 1 cup coconut milk
- ½ cup Greek yogurt
- 1 tablespoon almond butter
- 1 teaspoon vanilla extract

Instructions:

1. Place the banana, coconut milk, Greek yogurt, almond butter, and vanilla extract in the blender.
2. Blend until smooth and creamy.
3. Pour into a glass and enjoy the blissful combination of flavors.

Mango and Banana Smoothie

Ingredients:
- 1 cup mango chunks (fresh or frozen)
- 1 banana
- 1 cup almond milk (or any preferred milk)
- ½ cup plain yogurt
- 1 tablespoon honey (optional)

Instructions:
1. Add the mango chunks, banana, almond milk, and plain yogurt to the blender.
2. Blend until smooth and creamy.
3. Taste and add honey if additional sweetness is desired.
4. Serve immediately in a glass and enjoy the delightful tropical smoothie.

9. ANTIOXIDANT SMOOTHIES

Pomegranate Power

Ingredients:
- 1 cup pomegranate juice
- 1 banana
- 1 cup mixed berries (strawberries, blueberries, raspberries)
- ½ cup Greek yogurt
- 1 tablespoon honey (optional)

Instructions:
1. Add the pomegranate juice, banana, mixed berries, and Greek yogurt to the blender.
2. Blend until smooth and creamy.
3. Taste and add honey if additional sweetness is desired.
4. Pour into a glass and enjoy the antioxidant-rich smoothie.

Acai Berry Blast

Ingredients:
- 1 packet of frozen acai puree or 2 tablespoons acai powder
- 1 banana
- 1 cup mixed berries (fresh or frozen)
- 1 cup almond milk
- 1 tablespoon chia seeds (optional)

Instructions:
1. Combine the acai puree or powder, banana, mixed berries, and almond milk in the blender.
2. Blend until well combined and smooth.
3. If using, add chia seeds and blend briefly to mix.
4. Serve immediately in a glass and enjoy the berry blast.

Cherry and Berry Combo

Ingredients:
- 1 cup cherries (pitted, fresh or frozen)
- 1 cup mixed berries (strawberries, blueberries, blackberries)

- 1 banana
- 1 cup coconut water
- 1 tablespoon flaxseeds (optional)

Instructions:
1. Place the cherries, mixed berries, banana, and coconut water in the blender.
2. Blend until smooth and well combined.
3. If using, add flaxseeds and blend briefly to mix.
4. Pour into a glass and enjoy the delicious and healthy combo.

Cranberry Citrus Cooler

Ingredients:
- 1 cup cranberries (fresh or frozen)
- 1 orange, peeled and segmented
- 1 cup spinach (optional for added nutrients)
- 1 cup water
- 1 tablespoon honey (optional)

Instructions:

1. Add the cranberries, orange, spinach (if using), and water to the blender.
2. Blend until smooth and well combined.
3. Taste and add honey if additional sweetness is desired.
4. Serve immediately in a glass and enjoy the refreshing and tart cooler.

10. CALMING AND HEALING SMOOTHIES

Ginger Peach Smoothie

Ingredients:
- 1 cup peach slices (fresh or frozen)
- 1 banana
- 1 cup almond milk (or any preferred milk)
- 1-inch piece of fresh ginger, peeled and grated
- 1 tablespoon honey (optional)

Instructions:
1. Place the peach slices, banana, almond milk, and grated ginger in a blender.
2. Blend until smooth and creamy.
3. Taste and add honey if additional sweetness is desired.
4. Pour into a glass and enjoy the soothing ginger peach smoothie.

Chamomile and Honey Blend

Ingredients:
- 1 cup chamomile tea, cooled
- 1 banana
- 1 apple, cored and sliced
- 1 tablespoon honey
- ½ cup Greek yogurt

Instructions:
1. Brew a cup of chamomile tea and let it cool.
2. Combine the cooled chamomile tea, banana, apple slices, honey, and Greek yogurt in the blender.
3. Blend until smooth and well combined.
4. Serve immediately in a glass and enjoy the calming blend.

Aloe Vera and Mint Cooler

Ingredients:
- ½ cup aloe vera gel (fresh or store-bought)
- 1 cucumber, peeled and chopped
- 1 cup coconut water
- 1 tablespoon fresh mint leaves
- 1 tablespoon honey (optional)

Instructions:

1. Add the aloe vera gel, cucumber, coconut water, and mint leaves to the blender.
2. Blend until smooth and refreshing.
3. Taste and add honey if additional sweetness is desired.
4. Pour into a glass and enjoy the cool, healing smoothie.

Turmeric and Pineapple Elixir

Ingredients:
- 1 cup pineapple chunks (fresh or frozen)
- 1 banana
- 1 cup coconut milk
- 1 teaspoon ground turmeric
- 1 tablespoon honey (optional)

Instructions:

1. Combine the pineapple chunks, banana, coconut milk, and ground turmeric in the blender.
2. Blend until smooth and well combined.

3. Taste and add honey if additional sweetness is desired.
4. Serve immediately in a glass and enjoy the anti-inflammatory elixir.

11. SMOOTHIES FOR ENERGY AND VITALITY

Green Tea and Berry Blend

Ingredients:
- 1 cup brewed green tea, cooled
- 1 cup mixed berries (strawberries, blueberries, raspberries)
- 1 banana
- ½ cup Greek yogurt
- 1 tablespoon honey (optional)

Instructions:
1. Brew a cup of green tea and let it cool.
2. Combine the cooled green tea, mixed berries, banana, and Greek yogurt in the blender.
3. Blend until smooth and well combined.
4. Taste and add honey if additional sweetness is desired.
5. Serve immediately in a glass and enjoy the energizing blend.

Oatmeal and Banana Smoothie

Ingredients:
- 1 banana
- ½ cup rolled oats
- 1 cup almond milk (or any preferred milk)
- 1 tablespoon peanut butter or almond butter
- 1 teaspoon cinnamon
- 1 tablespoon honey (optional)

Instructions:
1. Place the banana, rolled oats, almond milk, peanut butter or almond butter, and cinnamon in the blender.
2. Blend until smooth and creamy.
3. Taste and add honey if additional sweetness is desired.
4. Pour into a glass and enjoy the hearty, energy-boosting smoothie.

Almond Butter and Blueberry Smoothie

Ingredients:
- 1 cup blueberries (fresh or frozen)

- 1 banana
- 1 cup almond milk
- 2 tablespoons almond butter
- 1 teaspoon vanilla extract

Instructions:

1. Combine the blueberries, banana, almond milk, almond butter, and vanilla extract in the blender.
2. Blend until smooth and creamy.
3. Serve immediately in a glass and enjoy the nutrient-dense smoothie.

Chia Seed and Raspberry Smoothie

Ingredients:
- 1 cup raspberries (fresh or frozen)
- 1 banana
- 1 cup coconut water
- 2 tablespoons chia seeds
- 1 tablespoon honey (optional)

Instructions:

1. Add the raspberries, banana, coconut water, and chia seeds to the blender.
2. Blend until smooth and well combined.
3. Taste and add honey if additional sweetness is desired.
4. Pour into a glass and enjoy the energy-boosting smoothie.

12. HIGH-PROTEIN SMOOTHIES

Greek Yogurt and Berry Boost

Ingredients:
- 1 cup mixed berries (strawberries, blueberries, raspberries)
- 1 cup Greek yogurt
- 1 banana
- 1 cup almond milk (or any preferred milk)
- 1 tablespoon honey (optional)

Instructions:
1. Place the mixed berries, Greek yogurt, banana, and almond milk in the blender.
2. Blend until smooth and creamy.
3. Taste and add honey if additional sweetness is desired.
4. Serve immediately in a glass and enjoy the protein-packed boost.

Peanut Butter and Banana Delight

Ingredients:
- 1 banana
- 2 tablespoons peanut butter
- 1 cup almond milk (or any preferred milk)
- ½ cup Greek yogurt
- 1 tablespoon chia seeds (optional)

Instructions:
1. Combine the banana, peanut butter, almond milk, and Greek yogurt in the blender.
2. Blend until smooth and creamy.
3. If using, add chia seeds and blend briefly to mix.
4. Pour into a glass and enjoy the creamy, protein-rich delight.

Cottage Cheese and Pineapple Smoothie

Ingredients:
- 1 cup pineapple chunks (fresh or frozen)
- ½ cup cottage cheese
- 1 banana
- 1 cup coconut water

- 1 tablespoon honey (optional)

Instructions:
1. Add the pineapple chunks, cottage cheese, banana, and coconut water to the blender.
2. Blend until smooth and creamy.
3. Taste and add honey if additional sweetness is desired.
4. Serve immediately in a glass and enjoy the refreshing, high-protein smoothie.

Protein-Packed Berry Blend

Ingredients:
- 1 cup mixed berries (strawberries, blueberries, raspberries)
- 1 scoop protein powder (vanilla or unflavored)
- 1 cup almond milk (or any preferred milk)
- ½ cup Greek yogurt
- 1 tablespoon flaxseeds (optional)

Instructions:
1. Combine the mixed berries, protein powder, almond milk, and Greek yogurt in the blender.

2. Blend until smooth and well combined.
3. If using, add flaxseeds and blend briefly to mix.
4. Serve immediately in a glass and enjoy the protein-packed berry goodness.

13. LOW-SUGAR SMOOTHIES

Cucumber and Mint Refresher

Ingredients:
- 1 cucumber, peeled and chopped
- 1 cup fresh mint leaves
- 1 cup water
- 1 tablespoon lemon juice
- ½ avocado (optional for creaminess)

Instructions:
1. Combine the cucumber, mint leaves, water, and lemon juice in the blender.
2. Blend until smooth and refreshing.
3. If using, add the avocado and blend again until creamy.
4. Serve immediately in a glass and enjoy the refreshing, low-sugar smoothie.

Avocado and Green Apple Smoothie

Ingredients:
- ½ avocado, peeled and pitted
- 1 green apple, cored and chopped
- 1 cup spinach
- 1 cup water or unsweetened almond milk
- 1 tablespoon lime juice

Instructions:
1. Place the avocado, green apple, spinach, and water (or almond milk) in the blender.
2. Blend until smooth and creamy.
3. Add lime juice and blend briefly to combine.
4. Pour into a glass and enjoy the creamy, low-sugar smoothie.

Celery and Melon Mix

Ingredients:
- 1 cup chopped celery
- 1 cup honeydew melon chunks
- 1 green apple, cored and chopped
- 1 cup water
- 1 tablespoon lemon juice

Instructions:
1. Combine the celery, honeydew melon, green apple, and water in the blender.
2. Blend until smooth and well combined.
3. Add lemon juice and blend briefly.
4. Serve immediately in a glass and enjoy the light, refreshing smoothie.

Carrot and Orange Cooler

Ingredients:
- 1 cup chopped carrots (raw or steamed)
- 1 orange, peeled and segmented
- 1 cup water or unsweetened almond milk
- 1 teaspoon ginger (optional for extra flavor)

Instructions:
1. Add the carrots, orange segments, and water (or almond milk) to the blender.
2. Blend until smooth and well combined.
3. If using, add ginger and blend briefly.
4. Pour into a glass and enjoy the cooling, low-sugar smoothie.

14. DETOX SMOOTHIES

Beet and Berry Cleanser

Ingredients:
- 1 small beet, peeled and chopped
- 1 cup mixed berries (strawberries, blueberries, raspberries)
- 1 apple, cored and chopped
- 1 cup water or unsweetened almond milk
- 1 tablespoon lemon juice

Instructions:
1. Combine the beet, mixed berries, apple, and water (or almond milk) in the blender.
2. Blend until smooth and well combined.
3. Add lemon juice and blend briefly.
4. Serve immediately in a glass and enjoy the vibrant detox smoothie.

Green Detox Smoothie

Ingredients:

- 1 cup spinach
- 1 cucumber, peeled and chopped
- 1 green apple, cored and chopped
- 1 cup coconut water
- 1 tablespoon lime juice

Instructions:
1. Place the spinach, cucumber, green apple, and coconut water in the blender.
2. Blend until smooth and well combined.
3. Add lime juice and blend briefly.
4. Pour into a glass and enjoy the refreshing green detox smoothie.

Lemon and Ginger Flush

Ingredients:
- 1 lemon, peeled and segmented
- 1-inch piece of fresh ginger, peeled and grated
- 1 cucumber, peeled and chopped
- 1 cup water
- 1 tablespoon honey (optional)

Instructions:

1. Combine the lemon, ginger, cucumber, and water in the blender.
2. Blend until smooth and well combined.
3. Taste and add honey if additional sweetness is desired.
4. Serve immediately in a glass and enjoy the cleansing flush.

Parsley and Pineapple Purifier

Ingredients:
- 1 cup fresh parsley leaves
- 1 cup pineapple chunks (fresh or frozen)
- 1 cucumber, peeled and chopped
- 1 cup water or coconut water
- 1 tablespoon lime juice

Instructions:
1. Place the parsley, pineapple chunks, cucumber, and water (or coconut water) in the blender.
2. Blend until smooth and well combined.
3. Add lime juice and blend briefly.

4. Pour into a glass and enjoy the purifying smoothie.

15. SEASONAL SMOOTHIES

Spring: Strawberry and Spinach Smoothie

Ingredients:
- 1 cup strawberries (fresh or frozen)
- 1 cup spinach
- 1 banana
- 1 cup almond milk (or any preferred milk)
- 1 tablespoon honey (optional)

Instructions:
1. Combine the strawberries, spinach, banana, and almond milk in the blender.
2. Blend until smooth and well combined.
3. Taste and add honey if additional sweetness is desired.
4. Serve immediately in a glass and enjoy the fresh taste of spring.

Summer: Watermelon and Mint Cooler

Ingredients:

- 2 cups watermelon chunks (fresh or frozen)
- 1 tablespoon fresh mint leaves
- 1 lime, juiced
- 1 cup water or coconut water
- 1 tablespoon honey (optional)

Instructions:
1. Place the watermelon chunks, mint leaves, lime juice, and water (or coconut water) in the blender.
2. Blend until smooth and refreshing.
3. Taste and add honey if additional sweetness is desired.
4. Pour into a glass and enjoy the cooling summer smoothie.

Fall: Pumpkin and Apple Spice

Ingredients:
- 1 cup pumpkin puree (canned or cooked)
- 1 apple, cored and chopped
- 1 cup almond milk (or any preferred milk)
- 1 teaspoon pumpkin pie spice
- 1 tablespoon maple syrup (optional)

Instructions:

1. Add the pumpkin puree, apple, almond milk, and pumpkin pie spice to the blender.
2. Blend until smooth and well combined.
3. Taste and add maple syrup if additional sweetness is desired.
4. Serve immediately in a glass and enjoy the cozy fall flavors.

Winter: Cranberry and Orange Smoothie

Ingredients:
- 1 cup cranberries (fresh or frozen)
- 1 orange, peeled and segmented
- 1 banana
- 1 cup water or almond milk
- 1 tablespoon honey (optional)

Instructions:

1. Combine the cranberries, orange segments, banana, and water (or almond milk) in the blender.
2. Blend until smooth and well combined.

3. Taste and add honey if additional sweetness is desired.

4. Pour into a glass and enjoy the bright, winter smoothie.

16. SPECIAL DIET SMOOTHIES

Gluten-Free Smoothies

Ingredients:
- 1 cup frozen mixed berries (strawberries, blueberries, raspberries)
- 1 banana
- 1 cup almond milk (or any preferred gluten-free milk)
- 1 tablespoon chia seeds
- 1 tablespoon honey (optional)

Instructions:
1. Place the mixed berries, banana, almond milk, and chia seeds in the blender.
2. Blend until smooth and well combined.
3. Taste and add honey if additional sweetness is desired.
4. Serve immediately in a glass and enjoy the gluten-free smoothie.

Vegan Smoothies

Ingredients:
- 1 cup frozen mango chunks
- 1 banana
- 1 cup coconut milk
- 1 tablespoon flaxseeds
- 1 tablespoon maple syrup (optional)

Instructions:
1. Combine the mango chunks, banana, coconut milk, and flaxseeds in the blender.
2. Blend until smooth and creamy.
3. Taste and add maple syrup if additional sweetness is desired.
4. Pour into a glass and enjoy the vegan-friendly smoothie.

Dairy-Free Smoothies

Ingredients:
- 1 cup frozen pineapple chunks
- 1 cup spinach
- 1 banana

- 1 cup almond milk
- 1 tablespoon hemp seeds

Instructions:
1. Add the pineapple chunks, spinach, banana, almond milk, and hemp seeds to the blender.
2. Blend until smooth and creamy.
3. Serve immediately in a glass and enjoy the dairy-free smoothie.

Low-FODMAP Smoothies

Ingredients:
- 1 cup spinach
- 1 small banana (unripe)
- 1 cup lactose-free almond milk
- 1 tablespoon chia seeds
- ½ cup blueberries (fresh or frozen)

Instructions:
1. Combine the spinach, banana, almond milk, chia seeds, and blueberries in the blender.
2. Blend until smooth and well combined.

3. Serve immediately in a glass and enjoy the low-FODMAP smoothie.

17. TIPS FOR MANAGING GASTROPARESIS

Dietary and Lifestyle Tips

1. Eat Small, Frequent Meals: Consuming smaller portions more frequently throughout the day can help prevent overwhelming your stomach and ease digestion.

2. Choose Low-Fiber Foods: High-fiber foods can be difficult to digest. Opt for low-fiber options like refined grains, well-cooked vegetables, and tender meats.

3. Focus on Soft, Easy-to-Digest Foods: Foods that are pureed, blended, or well-cooked are often easier to digest. Smoothies, soups, and stews can be beneficial.

4. Chew Food Thoroughly: Chewing food well breaks it down into smaller pieces, which can aid digestion and reduce stress on the stomach.

5. Avoid Lying Down After Eating: Wait at least 1-2 hours after eating before lying down to help reduce symptoms like nausea and bloating.

Foods to Avoid

1. High-Fiber Foods: Foods such as whole grains, nuts, seeds, and raw fruits and vegetables can be difficult to digest and may exacerbate symptoms.

2. Fatty Foods: Foods high in fat, like fried foods, fatty meats, and creamy sauces, can slow digestion and worsen symptoms.

3. Carbonated Beverages: Sodas and other fizzy drinks can cause bloating and gas, which may aggravate symptoms.

4. Spicy Foods: Spicy or heavily seasoned foods can irritate the stomach lining and contribute to discomfort.

5. Large Meals: Eating large meals can overwhelm the digestive system and lead to worsening symptoms. Smaller, more frequent meals are preferable.

Importance of Hydration

1. Stay Hydrated: Drink plenty of fluids throughout the day. Water, herbal teas, and clear broths are good choices.

2. Hydrate Between Meals: Drinking fluids between meals rather than with meals can help prevent feeling too full and support digestion.

3. Avoid Sugary and Caffeinated Beverages: These can lead to dehydration and may worsen symptoms. Stick to water and non-caffeinated herbal teas.

Working with Healthcare Providers

1. Regular Consultations: Schedule regular visits with your healthcare provider to manage symptoms, adjust treatment plans, and monitor progress.

2. Consult a Dietitian: A registered dietitian can help you create a personalized eating plan that meets your nutritional needs while accommodating your condition.

3. Medication Management: Discuss any prescribed medications with your healthcare provider to ensure they are effective and appropriate for your symptoms.

4. Monitor Symptoms: Keep a food and symptom diary to identify potential triggers and discuss findings with your healthcare team for better management of your condition.

18. CONCLUSION

Final Thoughts

Managing gastroparesis can be challenging, but with the right approach to diet and lifestyle, it is possible to alleviate symptoms and improve quality of life. This cookbook offers a variety of smoothie recipes designed to be gentle on the digestive system while providing essential nutrients. Remember, individual needs can vary, so use these recipes as a starting point and adjust based on your personal tolerance and preferences.

Encouragement for the Journey Ahead

Embarking on a journey to manage gastroparesis requires patience and persistence. Celebrate small victories and progress, and don't be discouraged by setbacks. Consistent efforts in making dietary and lifestyle changes can lead to meaningful improvements. Reach out to support networks, and stay positive about the steps you're taking to manage your condition.

Additional Resources

1. Gastroparesis Support Groups: Connecting with others who have similar experiences can provide support, advice, and encouragement. Online forums and local support groups can be valuable resources.

2. Registered Dietitians: Consulting with a dietitian who specializes in gastrointestinal disorders can offer personalized guidance and meal planning tailored to your needs.

3. Medical Websites: Reputable health websites like the American Gastroenterological Association (AGA) and the National Institute of Diabetes and Digestive and Kidney Diseases (NIDDK) offer valuable information about gastroparesis.

4. Books and Cookbooks: There are additional resources and cookbooks available that focus on managing gastroparesis through diet. These can offer further recipes and tips for navigating your dietary needs.

5. Healthcare Providers: Always consult your healthcare provider for tailored advice and treatment options. They can help you navigate the complexities of gastroparesis and work with you to create a comprehensive management plan.

www.ingramcontent.com/pod-product-compliance
Lightning Source LLC
Chambersburg PA
CBHW051657250726

48653CB00007B/2708